Easy

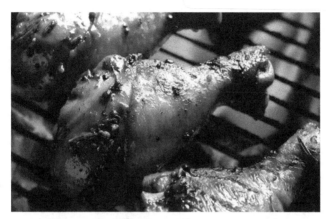

Delicious
Chicken Recipes

Improve your health and detox your body, with this mouth-watering and meat-based ideas. Use this cookbook for beginners to gain muscles and lose fat, getting a high-protein supply into your lifestyle and, furthermore, keeping a low budget

Dorian Gravy

2

Table of Contents

Welcome, dear hungry buddy!

This is my offer to your cooking style.

This cookbook is the realization of my research on how to eat tasty and healthy food at the meantime.
My purpose is to increase your energies and to let you live a lighter life, without the junk of the globalised kitchen.

In here, you'll find my knowledge on how to create delicious dishes with chicken.

Jump into a worldwide discovery of good food and natural-feed animals, with many recipes for a varied diet.

Nevertheless, you'll learn new techniques, discover tastes of all around the world and improve your skills.
Let yourself be inspired by the worldwide traditions, twisted by a proper chef.

Each of these dishes is thought to:

1 – Let you understand how to work with the meat of chicken

This majestic animal is presented in various dishes of different cultures, to show you how the same ingredient can change from dish to dish.

2 – Balance your weight with different cooking methods

As soon as you learn different ways to cook your meat, you'll discover an entire world of new ideas.
Chicken will never bore you again!

3 – Amaze your friends starting from the smell

Once your friends will come to dinner, they will be in love with your food even before to see your creation.

Chicken Recipes

"A chicken has feet and wings
Without finger things.
They cluck
And cannot pluck"

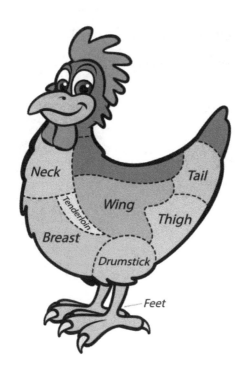

Caesar Salad Wraps

Serves 4 pax

Ingredients

- 4x 10" Low-carb tortillas
- 4 cups Romaine lettuce
- 3 Tbsp Parmesan cheese
- 3 Tbsp Light Caesar salad dressing
- 1.5 cup Cooked chicken

Procedure

1. Mix the chicken, salad dressing, cheese, and lettuce in a large bowl, tossing until the salad dressing evenly coats everything.
2. Spread out the tortillas and top each one with a heaping 1 cup of the salad.
3. Fold the sides in until they touch, then roll up from the bottom to make a wrap.
4. Wraps have all the benefits of a sandwich without all the carbs.
5. These are easy to prepare and require no cooking.

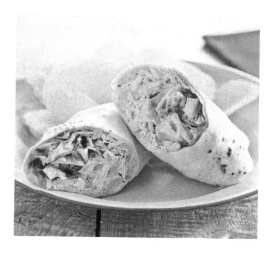

Avocado Stuffed Chicken

Serves 4 pax

Ingredients

- 0.25 tsp Black pepper
- 0.25 tsp Chili powder
- 0.25 tsp Ground cumin
- 0.5 tsp Garlic powder
- 1 cup Breadcrumbs
- 3 large Egg whites
- 0.25 tsp Salt
- 1 tsp Lime juice
- 1 Avocado
- 4x6 oz Boneless, skinless chicken breasts
- 9x13" baking dish coated with nonstick spray

Procedure

1. Set the oven temperature at 400° Fahrenheit.
2. Cut the avocado in half and scoop the flesh into a bowl; discard the skin and pit.
3. Mash the flesh with salt and lime juice. Spread a thin layer of avocado on each chicken breast.
4. Roll each breast across the width, securing the seams with toothpicks.
5. Beat the egg whites in a shallow mixing dish.
6. In another shallow mixing dish, combine the breadcrumbs with the chili powder, garlic powder, pepper, and cumin.
7. Carefully roll the stuffed chicken breasts in the egg white, then roll each in the breadcrumb mixture, pressing to coat.
8. Place the chicken breasts seam side down in the prepared dish.
9. Bake until the chicken is at least 165° Fahrenheit inside and the breadcrumbs are golden brown and crispy (30 min.).

Chicken Casserole

Serves 8 pax

Ingredients

- 0.75 cups Cheese, such as cheddar, mozzarella, or Gruyère
- 2.5 cups Cream of mushroom or broccoli soup
- 3.5 cups Non-starchy vegetables, such as asparagus, zucchini, or broccoli
- 0.25 tsp Salt
- 3 cups Chicken breasts
- 2.5 cups Quinoa, farro, brown rice, or other cooked grain

Procedure

1. Spread the grain in a 2 qt. baking dish and break the chicken over the top.
2. Top the chicken with the vegetables and the salt. Pour the soup over the vegetables, then sprinkle the cheese over everything.
3. Bake at 375°F until hot, about 30 minutes.
4. Serve hot.

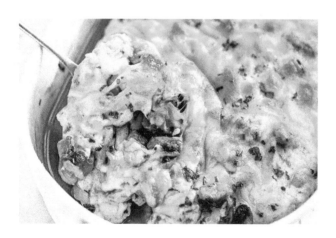

Cuban Sandwich

Serves 2 pax

Ingredients

- 1.5 oz Low sodium ham
- 1.5 oz Low-fat Swiss cheese
- 1.5 oz Low sodium turkey
- 2 oz Avocado
- 1 Multigrain pita

Procedure

1. Warm the oven to reach 350° Fahrenheit. Prep a baking tray using a layer of parchment baking paper.
2. Arrange the pita on it with cut sides facing up. Stack the cheese, avocado, turkey, and ham evenly on the bread pieces. Bake for 12 minutes.
3. Transfer it to the countertop and place the two halves of the bread together, forming one sandwich.
4. Warm a medium nonstick pan using the medium temperature setting.
5. Arrange the sandwich in the pan, holding it down with a spatula or heavy plate for two to three minutes.
6. Flip the sandwich and continue cooking for two to three minutes on the second side.
7. Cut in half and serve.

Chicken and Zucchini Enchiladas

Serves 6 pax

Ingredients

- 2 tsp Chili powder
- 0.25 cups Cilantro
- 0.5 tsp Dried oregano
- 1 cup Cheddar and Monterey jack cheese blend
- 3 cups Chicken, shredded and cooked
- 1 Onion
- 4 Zucchini
- 2 Garlic cloves
- 1.33 cupsGreen enchilada sauce
- 2 tsp Ground cumin
- 4 oz Hatch chili peppers
- 1 Tbsp Olive oil

Procedure

1. Prepare your oven to 350 F. Then, set a pan on the stovetop with your oil, warming it to medium-high.
2. Toss your onion in until the onion is translucent. Then, toss in garlic, chili powder, oregano, and cumin.
3. Toss in your shredded chicken, 1 cup of the enchilada sauce, and the green chilies.
4. Using a mandolin, slice your zucchini into thin sheets.
5. Overlap 3 slightly to create your roll, then place a dollop of chicken in the middle.
6. Roll the sheets and place them into your casserole dish. Repeat until you've used all of the chicken and zucchini.
7. Dump the rest of your enchilada sauce over the rolls, then cover the top with a light coat of cheese.
8. Bake for 20 minutes and serve garnished with cilantro.

Stuffed Chicken Breast

Serves 4 pax

Ingredients

- 4 Garlic cloves
- 4 Artichoke hearts
- 4 Chicken breasts
- 4 oz Low-fat mozzarella
- 1 tsp Paprika
- 1 tsp Curry powder
- 20 Basil leaves
- A pinch of pepper
- 4 tsp Sun-dried tomato

Procedure

1. Set your oven to 365 F.
2. Then, halfway through the breasts, slice through the lengthwise, creating a pocket in the breast.
3. Chop your basil, tomato, garlic, mozzarella, and artichoke. Combine well.
4. Stuff the breasts with the mixture.
5. Take toothpicks to close the chicken and hold it in place.
6. Place your chicken on top of a foil-lined sheet pan, then top with pepper, paprika, and curry powder.
7. Bake for 20 minutes, check the internal temperature, and when hot enough, serve alongside some veggies, quinoa, or other desired sides.
8. Serve.

Teriyaki Chicken Salad

Serves 6 pax

Ingredients

- 6 Bibb lettuce leaves
- 0.25 cups Slivered almonds
- 2 Celery
- 1 Carrot
- 3.75 cups Chicken breasts - cooked and shredded
- 0.25 cups Light mayonnaise
- 0.25 cups Plain, nonfat Greek yogurt
- 1 Tbsp Honey
- 1 Tbsp Splenda
- 1 Garlic clove
- 3 Tbsp Reduced-sodium soy sauce
- 0.25 cups Water

Procedure

1. Combine the honey, Splenda, water, soy sauce, and garlic in a saucepan using the high-temperature setting.
2. Wait until the mixture starts boiling, stirring occasionally, and adjust the temperature to med-low. Simmer until the sauce is reduced to 0.25 cups, about 8 minutes. Set aside to cool.
3. Once cooled, add the sauce to a large bowl. Mix in the yogurt and mayonnaise. Stir and add the chicken, carrots, celery, and almonds until thoroughly combined.
4. Place 0.75 cups of chicken salad in each lettuce leaf.

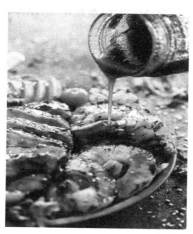

Chicken Pizza

Serves 1 pizza

Ingredients

- 1 cup chopped cilantro leaves
- 1 medium carrot, peeled and crudely grated
- 2 whole boneless, skinless chicken breasts, cut in half
- 1 unbaked pizza crust
- 1 cup bean sprouts
- 1 cup fontina cheese
- 4 green onions, trimmed and thinly cut
- 1/4 cup peanut or hot chili oil
- 1/2 cup crudely chopped dry-roasted peanuts
- 1 recipe Asian Marinade
- 1 cup mozzarella cheese

Procedure

1. Put the chicken breasts in an ovenproof dish. Pour the marinade over the chicken, flipping to coat completely. Cover and place in your fridge for minimum 8 hours.
2. Allow the chicken to return to room temperature before proceeding.
3. Preheat your oven to 325 degrees. Bake the chicken for thirty to forty minutes or until thoroughly cooked. Take away the chicken from the oven and let cool completely.
4. Shred the chicken into minuscule pieces; set aside.
5. Prepare the pizza dough in accordance with package directions.
6. Brush the dough with some of the oil. Top the oil with the cheeses, leaving a 1/2 inch rim.
7. Evenly spread the chicken, green onions, carrot, bean sprouts, and peanuts on top of the cheese. Sprinkle a little oil over the top.
8. Bake in accordance with package directions for the crust.
9. Remove from oven, drizzle with cilantro, serve.

Hot Wings and Cilantro Dip

Serves 4 pax

Ingredients

- 0.25 cups Cilantro
- 1 cup Plain nonfat Greek yogurt
- 0.5 tsp Black pepper
- Juice from one lime
- 1 tsp Thai style chili garlic sauce
- 1 Tbsp Soy sauce
- 1 Tbsp Garlic
- 0.5 cups No-sugar-added apricot preserves
- 2 lbs Chicken wing, skin removed

Procedure

1. Lay the chicken wings in a single layer on a baking tray coated with nonstick spray.
2. Lightly spray the wings with nonstick spray. Bake at 375°F for ten minutes.
3. Meanwhile, mix the apricot preserves, soy sauce, 2.5 tsp. of garlic, chili garlic sauce, 1 Tbsp. lime juice, and 0.25 tsp. black pepper.
4. After the wings have baked 10 minutes, spread them with the apricot sauce, then bake until the wings are cooked and the glaze is caramelized, about another 15 minutes.
5. Mix the Greek yogurt, lime juice (1 Tbsp.), 0.25 tsp. black pepper, and cilantro.
6. Serve the hot wings with the cilantro dip.

Stir-Fried Chicken

Serves 4 pax

Ingredients

- 2 Tbsp Soy sauce - low-sodium
- 1 Tbsp Olive oil
- 1 cup Chicken broth
- 2 tsp Corn starch
- 0.5 tsp Black pepper
- 1.5 cups Cooked chicken breast
- 1 Garlic clove
- 1x14 oz. bag Frozen stir-fry vegetables

Procedure

1. Prepare a nonstick skillet using the high temperature setting.
2. Mince the garlic. Cook the frozen vegetables in the oil (5-7 min.).
3. Meanwhile, mix the broth, soy sauce, corn starch, garlic, and black pepper.
4. Stir the sauce and the chicken into the pan and cook until the sauce is thick and the chicken is hot, about another 5 to 7 minutes.
5. Cool it thoroughly to store in a closed container up to seven days or serve immediately.

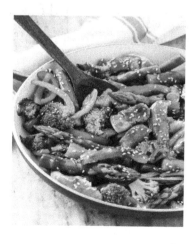

Bell Pepper Poppers

Serves 12 pax

Ingredients

- 1 Tbsp Parmesan cheese
- 1 Garlic clove, minced
- 1 slice Whole wheat bread, toasted
- 0.25 tsp Red pepper flakes
- 2 oz Soft goat cheese
- 4 oz Fat-free cream cheese
- 0.5 cup Onion, diced
- 2 slices Turkey bacon, chopped fine
- 12 Mini sweet peppers, sliced in half lengthwise

Procedure

1. Prepare the bacon in a nonstick skillet using the medium temperature setting until it's done and crispy.
2. Arrange it on paper towels to drain. In the same pan, cook the onions until translucent, stirring occasionally. Set aside.
3. Combine the goat and cream cheese. Mix in the onions, bacon, and pepper flakes.
4. Toss the toast, parmesan cheese, and garlic in a food processor. Pulse the mixture until it's thoroughly ground. Pour it into a small container and place it to the side for now.
5. Add 1 tsp. of cheese mixture in each pepper half. Press the cheese mixture side of the popper into the breadcrumbs mixture. Place on a baking sheet coated in nonstick spray.
6. Lightly spray the poppers using a spritz of nonstick spray.
7. Bake at 375°F until the breadcrumbs have turned a nice golden color and peppers have softened.
8. Serve

Chipolata Sausage

Serves 6 pax

Ingredients

- 1 tablespoon sage
- 1 teaspoon dried onion flakes
- 1 teaspoon thyme
- 7 pounds chicken butts
- 1 pound chicken fatback
- 1 teaspoon mace
- 6 ounces breadcrumbs
- 1 tablespoon pepper
- 1 pint water

Procedure

1. Grind the meat and fatback through a 3/8 plate. Mix the herbs and seasonings in the water and chill.
2. Purée the meat in a food processor and chill. Add the herbs, spices and seasonings to the meat. Add the breadcrumbs and chill the meat mixture. Set aside 12 ounces of mixture for the chipolata stuffing (recipe above).
3. Using 28mm casings, stuff the remaining mixture into 1-inch links and refrigerate. Grill, sauté or cook in the oven, as you prefer and serve at once.

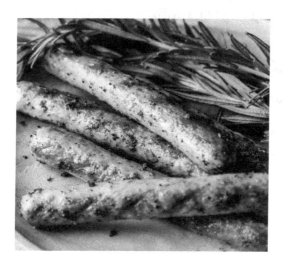

Sage Gravy

Serves 6 pax

Ingredients

- 1/4 cup finely chopped celery
- 1 tablespoon finely chopped fresh sage leaves
- 1/3 cup Chablis
- Reserved drippings (from capon recipe above).
- 1/2 cup finely chopped onion
- 1/2 cup finely chopped carrot
- 1/2 cup chicken broth
- 1/2 teaspoon pepper
- 1 tablespoon cold butter, cut into pieces
- 1 cup half-and-half (Equal parts milk and cream)
- 1/2 teaspoon lemon juice
- 1/2 teaspoon salt

Preparation

1. Mix onion, carrot, celery and chopped sage with drippings in a skillet. Cook on medium heat, stirring constantly, until onion is tender.
2. Add wine, bring to a boil, and cook until liquid reduces down to 2 tablespoons. Add broth and cook until liquid reduces by half.
3. Stir in half-and-half. Return to a boil. Cook until slightly thickened. Strain mixture through a wire-mesh into a bowl (discard vegetables).
4. Return mixture to skillet. Stir in lemon juice, salt, and pepper. Add butter, 1 piece at a time and stir with a wire whisk until fully blended.

Honey Chicken

Serves 6 pax

Ingredients

- 1 pound boneless, skinless chicken breasts, cut into bite-sized pieces
- 1/2 teaspoon Chinese 5-spice powder
- 1 (1-inch) piece ginger, peeled and minced
- 2 tablespoons vegetable oil
- 3 cloves garlic, thinly cut
- 1 medium onion, peeled and slice into wedges
- 2 tablespoons fish sauce
- 2 tablespoons honey
- 2 tablespoons soy sauce

Procedure

1. Mix the honey, fish sauce, soy sauce, and 5-spice powder in a small container; set aside.
2. Heat the oil in a wok on moderate to high. Put in the onion and cook until it just starts to brown.
3. Put in the chicken; stir-fry for three to four minutes.
4. Put in the garlic and ginger and continue stir-frying for 30 more seconds.
5. Mix in the honey mixture and allow to cook for three to four minutes, until the chicken is glazed and done to your preference.

Cajun Grains

Ingredients

- 15 oz. No-salt-added kidney beans
- 1 Tbsp Salt-free Cajun seasoning
- 1 White onion
- 1 Green bell pepper (1 medium, seeded)
- 8 oz 93% lean ground turkey
- 1 Tbsp Olive oil
- 15 oz Roasted diced tomatoes with green chiles
- 14.5 oz. can Chicken broth - Low sodium
- 0.5 tsp Salt
- 1 cup Whole farro

Ingredients

1. Drain and rinse the beans and farro in a colander. Dice/chop the bell pepper and onion.
2. In a medium saucepan, combine the farro, tomatoes with liquid, chicken broth, and salt.
3. Wait for it to boil using the high-temperature setting. Adjust the setting to med-low and simmer - covered (20 minutes).
4. Warm oil in a large nonstick skillet,using the med-high temperature setting.
5. Cook the turkey, onion, bell pepper, and Cajun seasoning in the oil until the turkey is cooked and the onion is translucent and softened (approx. 5 min.).
6. Mix the turkey mixture and beans into the saucepan with the farro, cover, and simmer for about 20 minutes, until the farro is tender.
7. Remove from heat and let rest, covered, for five minutes.

Chicken Satay

Serves 8 pax

Ingredients

- 0.25 cups Unsweetened coconut milk
- 2 Tbsp Peanut butter
- 2 clove Garlic
- 2 Tbsp Reduced-sodium soy sauce
- 2 Tbsp Brown sugar blend
- 0.5 tsp Sriracha
- 2 Tbsp Lime juice
- 1 tsp Fresh ginger
- 1 lb Boneless, skinless chicken breasts
- 8 Bamboo skewers

Procedure

1. Place the wood skewers in warm water for 1/2 of an hour. While they are soaking, slice the chicken breasts, lengthwise, into 8 strips.
2. Mix 1 Tbsp. Splenda, 1 minced garlic clove, 1 Tbsp. soy sauce, ginger, lime juice, and Sriracha in a medium mixing container. Place the chicken pieces in the marinade and refrigerate for 1 hour.
3. Preheat a grill. Use a small microwave-safe bowl to mix the peanut butter, coconut milk, 1 Tbsp. soy sauce, 1 Tbsp. Splenda, and remaining garlic.
4. Spear the chicken pieces on the bamboo skewers lengthwise, then grill for four to five minutes per side.
5. Microwave the sauce for 30 seconds, then stir again to thoroughly combine.
6. Serve the chicken with the dipping sauce on the side.

Tomato and Rice Pilaf

Ingredients

- 2 cloves garlic, minced
- 2 tablespoons extra virgin olive oil
- 3 cups chicken stock
- 2 teaspoons salt
- 4 teaspoons fresh ground black pepper
- 1/2 cup fresh basil, chopped
- 2 onions, chopped
- 4 pounds tomatoes, peeled, deseeded and chopped
- 1/2 teaspoon fresh ground cinnamon
- 8 cups basmati rice
- 1/2 cup toasted pine nuts

Instructions

1. Heat chicken stock to low simmer in medium saucepan.
2. Heat oil on medium low heat in large skillet. Add onions and garlic. Sauté until tender.
3. Add tomatoes and cinnamon. Cook 5 minutes on lowered heat. Add rice, stir well and cook 5 minutes.
4. Add simmering chicken stock. Stir until mixed. Cover and cook on low heat. Rice is cooked when tender and liquid is absorbed.
5. Remove from heat and let sit 5 minutes. Stir in salt, pepper, basil and pine nuts.
6. Serve.

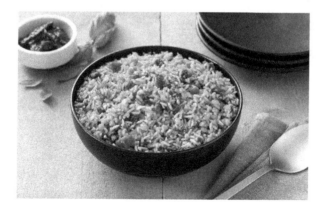

Jalapeño Chicken and Corns

Ingredients

- 1 Tbsp Olive oil
- 1 cup Nonfat Greek yogurt
- 2 cups Chicken breast
- 4 cups Chicken broth
- 0.5 tsp Black pepper
- 1 Tbsp Salt-free seasoning
- 4 cups Corn kernels
- 2 Garlic cloves
- 2 Jalapeño peppers
- 2 Carrots
- 1 Yellow onion
- 2 Celery stalks, chopped

Procedure

1. Peel and chop the garlic, carrots, and onion.
2. Prepare a Dutch oven or over-sized soup pot using the medium temperature setting to warm the oil.
3. Toss the celery, onion, carrots, jalapeños, corn, and garlic. into the pot to simmer for five to seven minutes.
4. Stir in the pepper, seasoning, and broth and bring to a boil. Adjust the temperature setting to a simmer for 20 minutes. Transfer the pan to a cool burner.
5. Puree about half of the soup, using a regular blender, food processor, or immersion blender. It might need to be done in batches.
6. Pour the puree back into the pot, then add the chicken and warm on medium until the chicken is hot.
7. Transfer the pan to the countertop, mix in the yogurt and serve immediately.

Sauced Supreme of Chicken

Ingredients

- 2 red bell peppers
- 2 green bell pepper
- 4 tablespoons butter
- Salt and freshly ground black pepper
- 1 lemon juice
- 8 chicken breasts
- 1 pound white button mushrooms
- 2 tomatoes, peeled and cut in quarters
- 1 cup dry sack sherry
- 1 sprig fresh parsley

Instructions

1. Season chicken with salt, pepper and lemon juice to taste. Cut peppers in half, top to bottom. Remove stem, seeds, and ribs. Slice peppers and set-aside.
2. Melt butter in skillet on medium high heat. Sauté chicken until golden brown. Remove chicken from skillet, set aside.
3. Add mushrooms and red wine to same skillet. Heat until wine reduces in half.
4. Return chicken breasts to skillet. Cover skillet and lower heat to a simmer Cook 10 minutes.
5. Add peppers and tomatoes. Heat uncovered until thoroughly warmed.
6. Garnish with parsley.
7. Serve on a bed of Rice Pilaf

Chicken Lettuce Wraps

Serves 3 pax

Ingredients

- 6 oz Grilled chicken
- 2 Tbsp Asian peanut sauce
- 6 Boston or Bibb lettuce leaves
- 2 Tbsp Julienne carrots
- 2 Scallion

Procedure

1. Lay two pieces of lettuce on each of 3 large plates. Place 1 oz. of chicken on top of each lettuce leaf and top the chicken with 1 tsp. peanut sauce each, 1 tsp. carrots, and then sprinkle the scallions over the carrots. Roll closed.
2. These high-protein wraps are low in carbs and are a fantastic method to use up leftover chicken.
3. The wraps come together very quickly and are also just plain delicious.

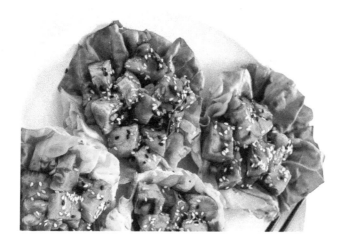

Chicken Flavored Pasta and Vegetables

Ingredients

- 0.5 cups Fat-free, low sodium chicken broth
- 8 oz Chickpea penne pasta
- 3 Tbsp Parmesan cheese
- 0.25 tsp Dried oregano
- 12 oz Broccoli florets
- 2 Zucchini
- 0.25 tsp Black pepper
- 0.5 tsp Salt
- 2 Tbsp Olive oil

Procedure

1. Set the oven at 400° Fahrenheit. Lightly spritz a baking tray using a cooking oil spray.
2. Prepare a large mixing container and add the zucchini, broccoli, salt, pepper, and oil.
3. Place mixture on the baking tray. Set a timer and bake for 20 minutes.
4. While the vegetables are cooking, cook the pasta by bringing water to a boil, then removing from heat and letting the pasta sit in the water for 4 to 6 minutes, stirring a few times. (Follow the directions on the package if you are uncertain.)
5. Drain the pasta, then add the chicken broth, cooked vegetables, and oregano; mix well. Top with parmesan cheese.
6. Serve immediately.

Crispy Baked Chicken

Serves 4 pax

Ingredients

- 4x5 oz Thin-sliced chicken cutlets
- 0.25 tsp Salt
- 0.75 tsp Adobo seasoning
- 0.5 cups Whole-wheat panko breadcrumb
- 2 Minced garlic cloves
- 0.5 tsp Dried oregano
- 1 tsp soy sauce - low-sodium
- 1 Egg white
- 2 Lime juice

Procedure

1. Prepare a baking tray using a spritz of cooking oil spray and heat it in a 425° Fahrenheit oven for ten minutes.
2. Mix the lime juice, egg white, soy sauce, oregano, and garlic in a medium-sized mixing container.
3. In a shallow dish, combine the panko, adobo seasoning, and salt.
4. Dip the chicken cutlets, one at a time, into the lime blend and then into the panko mixture, pressing so the crumbs stick.
5. Place the chicken on the hot baking tray, then lightly spray it with nonstick spray.
6. Set a timer and bake the chicken until the crust is golden and the chicken is fully cooked (20 min.).

Gluten-Free Chicken Salad Wraps

Serves 4 pax

Ingredients

- 4 cups Field greens
- 4 Gluten-free whole-grain wraps
- 0.25 tsp Dried thyme
- A pinch of Black pepper
- 3 Celery stalks, diced
- 2 Tbsp Hummus
- 0.25 cups Light mayonnaise
- 2 cups Cooked chicken breast

Procedure

1. Combine the chicken, celery, hummus, mayonnaise, thyme, and pepper in a medium mixing container.
2. Place 0.5 cups chicken salad in the center of each wrap. Place 1 cup field greens on top.
3. Fold the left and right side of each tortilla inward until they touch, then roll up from the bottom.
4. The whole grains and gluten-free wrap make this recipe a winner.
5. The hummus provides a nice contrast from more typical wraps, and these make a quick and easy meal.

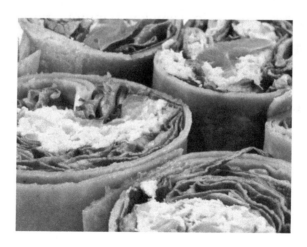

Chicken and Asparagus Rice

Serves 4 pax

Ingredients

- 2 cups Fresh asparagus tips or green beans
- 0.5 tsp Dried thyme
- 0.5 cups Reduced-fat sharp cheddar cheese
- 0.5 tsp Salt
- 8 oz Chicken thighs
- 2 cups Water
- 2 tsp Sodium-free chicken bouillon granules
- 4 Garlic cloves
- 1 cup Uncooked parboiled brown rice
- 1.5 cups Onion

Procedure

1. Remove the skin and bones from the chicken. Trim it into bite-sized pieces.
2. Coat a 3.5 to 4 qt. slow cooker with nonstick spray. Combine the water, chicken, onion, rice, garlic, bouillon, and thyme in the slow cooker and cook, covered, on high for 1.5 hours or low for 3 hours. Turn off the cooker.
3. Stir the rice with a fork. Mix in the asparagus or beans and let stand for about ten minutes. Mix in the salt and top with cheese.
4. Serve immediately.

Asian Chicken Stew

Serves 6 pax

Ingredients

- 2 Tbsp Hoisin sauce
- 1.5 cups Onion
- 1 cup Broccoli
- 2 tsp Crushed red pepper
- 2 Tbsp Soy sauce
- 1 cup Tomato juice
- 1/4 cup Green onions
- 1 Tbsp Peanut oil
- 1/2 cup Pickled cherry peppers
- 1 lb Pre-cooked chicken
- 1 tsp Sesame seeds

Procedure

1. Toss all ingredients, save for the green onion and sesame seeds, into a slow cooker. Stir to so everything is well mixed. Set the cooker to low, cover, and cook for two hours.
2. When serving, top bowls with green onion slices and sesame seeds.

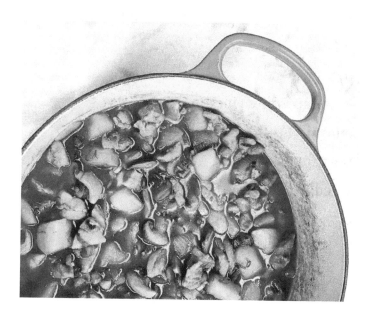

Gingered Garlic Chicken and Broccoli

Serves 4 pax

Ingredients

- 4 Garlic cloves, minced
- 4 Medjool dates
- 1 Broccoli head, florets
- 1 lb Chicken breast, boneless, skinless
- 0.25 cup Sesame oil
- 0.5 cup Water
- 0.25 cup White vinegar
- 2 inches Fresh ginger chunk
- 0.25 cup Olive oil
- 1 Red pepper
- 0.75 cup Reduced sodium soy sauce

Procedure

1. With your oven preheating to 425°F, take a medium bowl and mix together your water, garlic, oil, vinegar, ginger, soy sauce, and dates. Mix to combine well, then set aside.
2. Set up your other ingredients. Slice up your chicken into strips. Then, cut your broccoli into florets and bell pepper into julienne strips.
3. Place your chicken, bell pepper, and broccoli into a single layer on a baking sheet without touching.
4. Drizzle the dressing from earlier all over the chicken and veggies, reserving 1/2 c. of dressing. Bake for 10 minutes.
5. Boil the last 1/2 cup of dressing, dropping to a simmer and allowing it to thicken for 10 minutes.
6. When thick and chicken and veggies are done, pull them out and pour the chicken and veggies with the sauce.
7. Divide into four containers, topped with sesame seeds, green onions, and sesame oil.
8. Serve.

Chicken Broth

Serves 8 cups

Ingredients

- 1 onion, chopped
- 2 teaspoons salt
- 4 pounds chicken backs and wings
- 14 cups water
- 2 bay leaves

Procedure

1. Heat chicken and water in big stockpot or Dutch oven on moderate to high heat until boiling, skimming off any scum that comes to surface. Decrease heat to low and simmer slowly for three hours.

2. Put in onion, bay leaves, and salt and continue to simmer for another 2 hours.

3. Strain broth through fine-mesh strainer into a big container, pressing on solids to extract as much liquid as possible.

4. Allow broth to settle for approximately five minutes, then skim off fat.

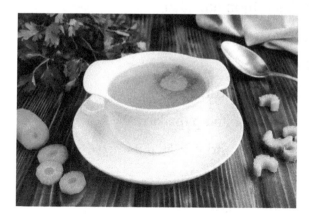

Chicken, Apples and Brussels Sprouts

Serves 2 pax

Ingredients

- 0.5 tsp Garlic powder
- A pinch of Salt
- A pinch of Black pepper
- 12 oz Boneless, skinless chicken thighs
- 0.5 tsp Sweet paprika
- 0.5 tsp Onion powder
- 1.5 Tbsp Spicy maple syrup
- 1 Tbsp Dijon mustard
- 4 Sage leaves
- 1 Apple
- 1 Purple top turnip
- 0.5 tsp Smoked paprika
- 0.5 tsp Ground yellow mustard
- 3 Carrots
- 4 oz Brussels sprouts

Procedure

1. Cut the stems off the Brussels sprouts, then cut them in quarters lengthwise. Peel the carrots, cut them in half lengthwise, cut crosswise into 2" pieces. Cut off the ends of the turnip, then chop it into medium pieces.

2. Prepare a large mixing container and mix the turnip, carrots, and Brussels sprouts. Core the apple and dice it into medium pieces. Remove the sage leaves from the stems, then thinly slice the leaves. Combine the mustard, maple syrup, and water in a bowl, mixing well. Stir in salt and pepper.

3. Cover a sheet pan with foil. In a small bowl, combine the ground yellow mustard, sweet paprika, garlic powder, smoked paprika, and onion powder. Add 0.5 tsp. of oil to the bowl of vegetables, then mix in the spice mixture. Toss to coat thoroughly.

4. Spread the vegetables on the prepared pan in an even layer and bake at 450°F until tender when pierced with a fork and lightly browned, 20 to 22 minutes. Remove from the oven.

5. Pat the chicken dry with paper towels. Dust it using pepper and salt and pepper. In a medium, nonstick pan over medium-high heat, heat 0.5 tsp. olive oil.

6. Cook the chicken until lightly browned, 6 to 8 minutes. Add the apple and cook for another 6 to 8 minutes, or until the chicken is fully cooked (at least 165° in the center) and the apple is softened. Move the cooked chicken to plates but leave the apple in the pan.

7. Stir the mustard sauce and sliced sage to the cooked apple in the pan. Cook on medium-high 30 seconds to 1 minute, stirring frequently, until the apple is thoroughly coated.

8. Remove from the heat and spoon over the chicken. Serve.

Moroccan Chicken Lentil Soup

Serves 8 pax

Ingredients

- 1/4 cup harissa, plus extra for serving
- 1/4 teaspoon ground cinnamon
- 1/3 cup minced fresh cilantro
- 1/2 teaspoon paprika
- 3/4 cup green or brown lentils
- 1 (15-ounce) can chickpeas, rinsed
- 1 onion, chopped fine
- 1 tablespoon all-purpose flour
- 1 tablespoon extra-virgin olive oil
- 1 teaspoon grated fresh ginger
- 1 teaspoon ground cumin
- 10 cups chicken broth
- 1 pound bone-in split chicken breasts, trimmed
- 4 plum tomatoes, cored and cut into pieces
- Pinch saffron threads, crumbled

Procedure

1. Pat chicken dry using paper towels and sprinkle with salt and pepper. Heat oil in Dutch oven on moderate to high heat until just smoking. Brown chicken lightly, approximately three minutes each side; move to plate.

2. Put in onion to fat left in pot and cook on moderate heat till they become tender, approximately five minutes.

3. Mix in ginger, cumin, paprika, cinnamon, cayenne, 1/4 teaspoon pepper, and saffron and cook until aromatic, approximately half a minute. Mix in flour and cook for about sixty seconds. Slowly beat in broth, scraping up any browned bits and smoothing out any lumps, and bring to boil.

4. Mix in lentils and chickpeas, then nestle chicken into pot and bring to simmer. Cover, decrease the heat to low, and simmer gently until chicken registers 160 degrees, fifteen to twenty minutes.

5. Move chicken to slicing board, allow to cool slightly, then shred into bite-size pieces using 2 forks, discarding skin and bones. In the meantime, continue to simmer lentils, covered, for 25 to 30 minutes.

6. Mix in shredded chicken and cook until heated through, approximately two minutes. Mix in tomatoes, cilantro, and harissa and sprinkle with salt and pepper to taste.

7. Serve, passing extra harissa separately.

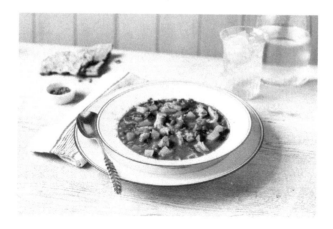

Spicy Chicken, Rice and Beans

Serves 5 pax

Ingredients

- 1 tsp Basil
- 1 (15 oz.) can Black beans
- 1 tsp Cayenne pepper
- 1 lb Chicken breast, skinless, boneless
- 1 tsp Chili powder
- 1 tsp Cumin
- 1 Garlic clove
- 1 tsp Garlic powder
- 3 tbsp Olive oil
- 1 tsp Oregano
- 1 cup Ric
- 15 oz Salsa
- Salt
- Water (1 c. and one-quarter c. separated)
- 2 Tbsp White vinegar

Procedure

1. Using a food processor or blender, process the olive oil, a quarter cup of water, oregano, garlic, basil, and vinegar. Sprinkle in salt and pepper and set aside.

2. In a bigger baking dish or container, combine your rice, salsa, and remaining water. Add a bit of oil and stir.

3. Slice the chicken breast into five equally sized pieces. Sprinkle the chili powder, garlic, and remaining seasonings on the chicken. Rub the spice blend throughout the chicken.

4. Place the chicken slices on the rice and salsa. Move the mixture into a pot and get it up to boiling. Once boiling, reduce heat, so the food simmers. Cover and cook until the rice and chicken are fully cooked.

5. Take out your chicken from your pot and leave it on the side.

6. Keeping the heat low, introduce black beans, the vinegar dressing made earlier, and a touch of oil.

7. Once warmed through, divide into five equal portions.

Chicken and Basil

Serves 4 pax

Ingredients

- 2 tablespoons soy sauce
- 2 teaspoons sugar
- 2 tablespoons fish sauce
- 1 big onion, cut into thin slices
- 1 tablespoon water
- 2 cups chopped basil leaves, divided
- cloves garlic, minced
- 3 Thai chilies, seeded and thinly cut
- 2 tablespoons vegetable oil
- 1 whole boneless, skinless chicken breasts, cut into 1-inch cubes

Procedure

1. In a moderate-sized-sized container, mix the fish sauce, the soy sauce, water, and sugar. Put in the chicken cubes and stir to coat. Let marinate for about ten minutes.

2. In a big frying pan or wok, heat oil on moderate to high heat. Put in the onion and stir-fry for two to three minutes. Put in the chilies and garlic and carry on cooking for another half a minute.

3. Using a slotted spoon, remove the chicken from the marinade and put in it to the frying pan (reserve the marinade.) Stir-fry until almost thoroughly cooked, approximately 3 minutes.

4. Put in the reserved marinade and cook for another half a minute. Take away the frying pan from the heat and mix in 1 cup of the basil.

5. Decorate using the rest of the basil and serve with rice.

Chicken and Brandy

Ingredients

- 1 whole roasting chicken, washed and trimmed of surplus fat
- 6 tablespoons soy sauce
- 1/4 cup vegetable oil
- 1 (1-inch) piece ginger, cut
- 1 teaspoon salt
- 8 cloves garlic, minced
- 2 shots brandy
- 2 tablespoons black soy sauce

Procedure

1. Fill a pot big enough to hold the whole chicken roughly full of water. Bring the water to its boiling point using high heat.

2. Lower the heat to moderate and cautiously put in the chicken to the pot. Regulate the heat so that the water is just simmering.

3. Poach the whole chicken for twenty minutes to half an hour or until thoroughly cooked. Cautiously remove the chicken from the pot, ensuring to drain the hot water from the cavity of the bird. Position the chicken aside to cool.

4. Take away the skin from the bird and discard. Take away the meat from the chicken and cut it into 1-inch pieces; set aside.

5. Put in the oil to a big frying pan or wok and heat on medium. Put in the soy sauces, salt, and garlic. Stir-fry until the garlic starts to tenderize, approximately half a minute to one minute.

6. Put in the chicken pieces, stirring to coat. Mix in the brandy and the ginger.

7. Cover the frying pan or wok, decrease the heat to low, and simmer five to ten more minutes.

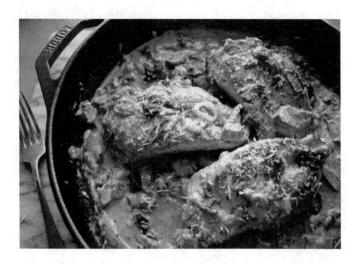

Red Pepper and Chicken

Serves 4 pax

Ingredients

- 1x15 oz Black beans
- Black pepper
- 1 Onion
- 4 Chicken breast halves
- 4 cups cooked rice or couscous
- 1x12 oz Roasted sweet red peppers
- 1x14.5 oz Mexican stewed tomatoes

Procedure

1. Set the chicken breasts into the crock of your slow cooker.
2. Dump in the beans, red peppers, onion, tomatoes, and black pepper over the chicken.
3. Cover and cook on low for six hours.
4. When done, serve on a bed of rice or couscous.

Chicken, Garlic and Black Pepper

Serves 4 pax

Ingredients

- 1 teaspoon sugar
- 2 pounds boneless, skinless chicken breasts, cut into strips
- 1 cup fish sauce
- 1 tablespoon whole black peppercorns
- 2 tablespoons vegetable oil
- 5 cloves garlic, cut in half

Procedure

1. Using either a mortar and pestle or a food processor, mix the black peppercorns with the garlic.
2. Put the chicken strips in a big mixing container. Put in the garlic-pepper mixture and the fish sauce and stir until blended.
3. Cover the container, place in your fridge, and let marinate for twenty minutes to half an hour.
4. Heat the vegetable oil on moderate heat in a wok or frying pan. When it is hot, put in the chicken mixture and stir-fry until thoroughly cooked, approximately 3 to five minutes.
5. Mix in the sugar. Put in additional sugar or fish sauce to taste.

Fried Spicy Chicken

Ingredients

- 1/2 teaspoon ground coriander
- 2 tablespoons vegetable oil
- 4 pounds chicken pieces, washed and patted dry
- 3 tablespoons Tamarind Concentrate
- 1/2 teaspoon white pepper
- 2 teaspoons salt, divided
- 2 small onions, thinly cut
- 8 big red chilies, seeded and chopped
- A pinch of turmeric
- Vegetable oil for deep-frying

Procedure

1. In a small container mix the tamarind, turmeric, coriander, 1 teaspoon of the salt, and the pepper.
2. Put the chicken pieces in a big Ziplock bag. Pour the tamarind mixture over the chicken, seal the bag, and marinate minimum 2 hours or overnight in your fridge.
3. In a small sauté pan, heat 2 tablespoons of vegetable oil on moderate heat. Put in the red chilies, onions, and the rest of the salt; sauté for five minutes. Set aside to cool slightly.
4. Move the chili mixture to a food processor and pulse for a short period of time to make a coarse sauce.
5. Drain the chicken and discard the marinade. Deep-fry the chicken pieces in hot oil until the skin is golden and the bones are crunchy. Take away the cooked chicken to paper towels to drain.
6. Put the cooked chicken in a big mixing container. Pour the chili sauce over the chicken and toss until each piece is uniformly coated.

Roasted Chicken

Serves 4 pax

Ingredients

For the marinade:

- 1/2 cup fish sauce
- 2 tablespoons crushed garlic
- 2 tablespoons freshly grated gingerroot
- 1/2 cup sweet dark soy sauce
- 1 tablespoon freshly ground black pepper

For the stuffing:

- 1/2 cup freshly grated ginger
- 1 roasting chicken, cleaned and patted dry
- 1/2 cup cut bruised lemongrass stalks
- 1/2 cup chopped cilantro
- 1/2 cup chopped mushrooms
- 1/2 cup fresh grated galangal

Procedure

1. Mix all of the marinade ingredients in a plastic bag big enough to hold the whole chicken.
2. Put in the chicken, ensuring to coat the whole bird with the marinade. Put the chicken in your fridge and leave overnight.
3. Take away the chicken from the plastic bag, saving for later the marinade.
4. Put all of the stuffing ingredients in a big mixing container. Mix in the reserved marinade.
5. Fill the bird's cavity and place it breast side up in a roasting pan.
6. Put the roasting pan in a preheated 400°F oven and roast for 50 to 60 minutes, or until the juices run clear.

Chicken and Ginger

Serves 2 pax

Ingredients

- 2 tablespoons dark soy sauce
- 2 tablespoons fish sauce
- 2 tablespoons oyster sauce
- 1 cup cut domestic mushrooms
- 1 tablespoon chopped garlic
- 1 whole boneless, skinless chicken breast, cut into bite-sized pieces
- 3 tablespoons vegetable oil
- 3 tablespoons Cilantro
- 2 cups Jasmine rice, cooked in accordance with package directions
- A pinch of sugar
- 2 habanero or bird's eye chilis
- 3 tablespoons chopped onion
- 3 tablespoons grated ginger

Procedure

1. In a small container mix the fish, soy, and oyster sauces; set aside.
2. Heat the oil in a big wok until super hot. Put in the garlic and chicken, and stir-fry just until the chicken starts to change color.
3. Put in the reserved sauce and cook until it starts to simmer while stirring continuously.
4. Put in the mushrooms, ginger, sugar, onion, and chilies; simmer until the chicken is thoroughly cooked, approximately eight minutes.
5. To serve, ladle the chicken over Jasmine rice and top with green onion and cilantro.

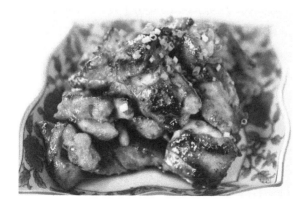

Wild Chicken

Serves 2 pax

Ingredients

- 10 basil leaves
- 2 (2-inch-long, 1/2-inch wide) strips of lime peel
- 2 tablespoons fish sauce
- 2 tablespoons vegetable oil
- 1/2 cup coconut milk
- 1 stalk lemongrass, inner portion roughly chopped
- 1 whole boneless, skinless chicken breast, cut into fine strips
- 2 serrano chilies, stems and seeds removed

Procedure

1. Put the chilies, lemongrass, and lime peel into a food processor and pulse until ground.
2. Heat the oil on moderate to high heat in a wok or big frying pan. Put in the chili mixture and sauté for one to two minutes.
3. Mix in the coconut milk and cook for a couple of minutes.
4. Put in the chicken and cook until the chicken is thoroughly cooked, approximately five minutes.
5. Decrease the heat to low and put in the fish sauce and basil leaves to taste.
6. Serve with sufficient Jasmine rice.

Red Hot Chili Chicken

Serves 2 pax

Ingredients

- 2 kaffir lime leaves or 2 (2-inch-long, 1/2–inch wide) pieces of lime zest
- 1 tablespoon basil leaves
- 2 tablespoons fish sauce
- 1 tablespoon vegetable oil
- 4 ounces Thai eggplant
- 1 tablespoons Red Curry Paste
- 1/2 cup coconut milk
- 1 whole boneless, skinless chicken breast, cut into bite-sized pieces
- 1 tablespoon brown sugar

Procedure

1. In a big frying pan or wok, heat the oil on moderate to high heat. Mix in the curry paste and cook until aromatic, approximately one minute.

2. Lower the heat to moderate-low and put in the coconut milk. Stirring continuously, cook until a thin film of oil develops on the surface.

3. Put in all of the rest of the ingredients except the eggplant. Bring to its boiling point, reduce heat, and simmer until the chicken starts to turn opaque, approximately five minutes.

4. Put in the eggplant and carry on cooking until the chicken is done to your preference, approximately 3 minutes more.

5. Serve.

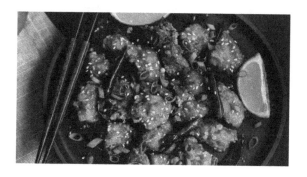

Twin Roasted Chicken

Serves 4 pax

Ingredients

- 1 clove garlic, minced
- 1 medium onion, chopped
- 1 tablespoon fish sauce
- 1 teaspoon dried red pepper flakes
- 1 whole roasting chicken
- 2 stalks lemongrass, thinly cut (soft inner core only)
- Salt and pepper to taste
- Vegetable oil

Procedure

1. To prepare the marinade, put the lemongrass, onion, garlic, red pepper, and fish sauce in a food processor. Process until a thick paste is formed. Place in your fridge for minimum 30 minutes, overnight if possible.

2. Spread the marinade throughout the chicken cavity and then drizzle the cavity with salt and pepper. Rub the outside of the bird with a small amount of vegetable oil (or butter if you prefer) and sprinkle with salt and pepper.

3. Put the bird in a roasting pan, and cover it using plastic wrap. Place in your fridge for a few hours to marinate, if possible.

4. Take away the chicken from the fridge roughly thirty minutes before roasting.

5. Preheat your oven to 500 degrees. Take away the plastic wrap and put the bird in your oven, legs first, and roast for 50 to 60 minutes or until the juices run clear.

6. Serve.

Chicken Sweet 'n Sour

Serves 4 pax

Ingredients

- 2 tablespoons soy sauce
- 4 tablespoons prepared Plum Sauce
- 1 (1-inch) piece of ginger, peeled and minced
- 1 green and 1 red bell pepper, seeded and slice into 1-inch pieces
- 1 tablespoon vegetable oil
- 8 ounces canned pineapple pieces, drained
- Jasmine rice, cooked in accordance with package directions
- 1 pound boneless, skinless chicken breasts, cut into 1-inch cubes
- 1 small onion, thinly cut
- 2 cloves garlic, minced
- 2 tablespoons prepared chili sauce

Procedure

1. In a small container, mix the soy sauce, garlic, ginger, and chili sauce. Put in the chicken pieces, stirring to coat. Set aside to marinate for minimum twenty minutes.

2. Heat the oil in a wok or big frying pan on moderate heat. Put in the onion and sauté until translucent, approximately 3 minutes.

3. Put in the chicken mixture and carry on cooking for another three to five minutes.

4. Put in the bell peppers, the pineapple, and plum sauce. Cook for another five minutes or until the chicken is thoroughly cooked.

5. Serve over lots of fluffy Jasmine rice.

Tamarind Chicken and Mushrooms

Serves 2 pax

Ingredients

- 4 ounces domestic mushrooms, cut
- 1/2 cup cut onions
- clove garlic, minced
- tablespoons Tamarind Concentrate
- 2 tablespoons vegetable oil
- Salt and freshly ground black pepper
- 1/4 cup chopped basil
- 2 whole boneless, skinless chicken breasts, cut into bite-sized cubes
- 1 teaspoon sugar
- 2 tablespoons water
- 1 cup bean sprouts
- 1 small jalapeño, seeded and minced

Procedure

1. Heat the vegetable oil in a big sauté pan or wok using high heat. Flavor the chicken with the salt, pepper, and sugar.
2. Put in the chicken to the pan and stir-fry for a couple of minutes. Put in the mushrooms, onions, and garlic; carry on cooking for another two to three minutes. Put in the tamarind and water; stir.
3. Put in the rest of the ingredients. Adjust seasonings to taste before you serve.

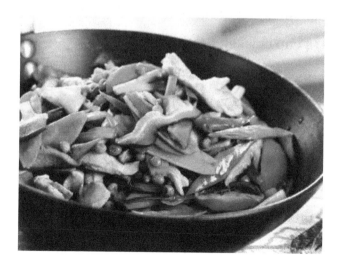

Cashew Thai Chicken

Serves 4 pax

Ingredients

- 3/4 cup whole cashews
- 3 teaspoons Chili Tamarind Paste
- 10 dried Thai chilies
- 10 cloves garlic, mashed
- 4 green onions, trimmed and slice into 1-inch lengths
- 1 small onion, thinly cut
- 1/4 cup chicken broth
- 1 tablespoon oyster sauce
- 3 tablespoons vegetable oil
- 1 big whole boneless, skinless chicken breast, cut into fine strips
- 1 tablespoon fish sauce
- 5 tablespoons sugar

Procedure

1. In a wok or big frying pan, heat the oil on moderate to high heat until hot.
2. Put in the chilies and stir-fry for a short period of time until they darken in color. Move the chilies to a paper towel to drain; set aside.
3. Put in the garlic to the wok and stir-fry until just starting to turn golden.
4. Increase the heat to high and put in the chicken. Cook while stirring continuously, for roughly one minute. Put in the green onions and onion slices and cook for half a minute.
5. Put in the Chili Tamarind Paste, broth, oyster sauce, fish sauce, and sugar. Continue to stir-fry for 30 more seconds.
6. Put in the reserved chilies and the cashews; stir-fry for 1 more minute or until the chicken is thoroughly cooked and the onions are soft.

Glazed Thai Chicken

Serves 4 pax

Ingredients

- 1 tablespoon fish sauce
- 2 tablespoons soy sauce
- 4 cloves garlic, chopped
- 1 teaspoon white pepper
- 1 whole chicken, cut in half
- 1 tablespoon minced cilantro
- 1 teaspoon chopped ginger
- 1 teaspoon salt
- 3 tablespoons coconut milk
- 2 tablespoons rice wine

Procedure

1. Wash the chicken under cold water, then pat dry. Trim off any surplus fat or skin. Put the chicken halves in big Ziplock bags.

2. Mix the rest of the ingredients together in a small container until well blended.

3. Pour the marinade into the Ziplock bags, seal closed, and turn until the chicken is uniformly coated with the marinade. Allow the chicken to marinate for thirty minutes to an hour in your fridge.

4. Preheat your oven to 350 degrees. Take away the chicken from the bags and put them breast side up in a roasting pan big enough to hold them easily. Roast the chicken for about forty-five minutes.

5. Turn on the broiler and broil for roughly ten minutes or until done.

Chicken and Lemongrass Skewers

Ingredients

- 2 teaspoons fish sauce
- 5 stalks lemongrass, trimmed
- 2 teaspoons Black pepper
- 2 teaspoons sugar
- Sea salt to taste
- 12 big cubes chicken breast meat, a little over 1 ounce each
- 2 tablespoons vegetable oil, divided
- Juice of 1 lime
- Pinch of dried red pepper flakes

Procedure

1. Remove 2 inches from the thick end of each stalk of lemongrass; set aside. Bruise 4 of the lemongrass stalks using the back of a knife. Take away the tough outer layer of the fifth stalk, exposing the soft core; mince.

2. Skewer 3 cubes of chicken on each lemongrass stalk. Drizzle the skewers with the minced lemongrass and black pepper, and sprinkle with 1 tablespoon of oil. Cover using plastic wrap and place in your fridge for twelve to one day.

3. Chop all of the reserved lemongrass stalk ends. Put in a small deep cooking pan and cover with water. Bring to its boiling point, cover, and let reduce until roughly 2 tablespoons of liquid is left; strain. Return the liquid to the deep cooking pan and further reduce to 1 tablespoon.

4. Mix the lemongrass liquid with the red pepper flakes, lime juice, fish sauce, sugar, and remaining tablespoon of oil; set aside.

5. Prepare a grill to high heat. Grill the chicken skewers for roughly two to three minutes per side, or until done to your preference.

6. To serve, spoon a little of the lemongrass sauce over the top of each skewer and drizzle with sea salt.

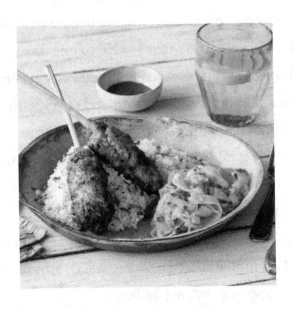

Bonus Risotto Recipes

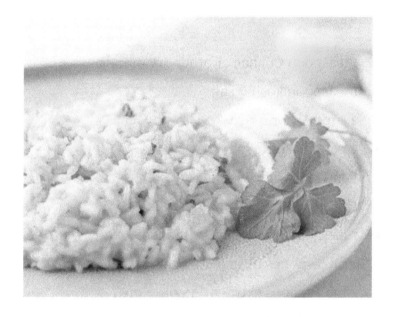

Cuttlefish Risotto

Serves 4 pax

Ingredients

- 1 teaspoon Cognac or other dry brandy
- 1 teaspoon kosher salt
- 2 cups Arborio rice
- 2 pounds cuttlefish
- 1 cup dry white wine
- 1 garlic clove, finely chopped
- 1 medium onion, finely chopped
- 2 tablespoons unsalted butter, cut into pieces
- 3 tablespoons extra-virgin olive oil
- 6 cups Fish Stock
- Freshly ground black pepper

Procedure

1. In a moderate-sized deep cooking pan, bring the stock to a bare simmer. Clean the cuttlefish by removing the blade-shaped interior cartilage, skin, and innards, saving for later two of the ink sacs. (Two ink sacs are enough for this dish; the others can be frozen.)

2. With a mortar and pestle, work the contents of the sac until the desired smoothness is achieved, discarding the actual sacs, or work in a small chopper with ⅓ cup of water, and save for later.

3. Pull and separate the head and tentacles from the body. Chop off the tentacles, discarding the eyes, and squeeze out the cartilage mouth from the center of the tentacles and discard. Quarter the tentacles along the length.

4. Chop the body into ½-inch strips. Rinse the bodies and tentacles and drain.

5. In a big straight-sided frying pan on moderate heat, heat the olive oil. Once the oil is hot, put in the onion, and cook, stirring once in a while, until translucent, approximately three minutes.

6. Put in the garlic, and sauté until aromatic but not browned, one minute. Put in the cuttlefish, and flavor with the salt and some black pepper.

7. Sauté until the cuttlefish exudes its liquid, approximately five minutes. Put in the wine and 1 cup stock. Simmer, covered, until the cuttlefish is soft, half an hour, putting in slightly more stock, if required, to keep the cuttlefish covered in liquid while cooking.

8. Put in the rice and regulate the heat so the liquid is simmering. Simmer until the rice absorbs all of the liquid in the pan. Mix in the cuttlefish ink.

9. Gradually put in more hot stock as the previous additions have been absorbed, stirring all the while, until the rice is firm to the bite and the risotto is creamy, eighteen minutes from the addition of the rice. (You may not need to use all of the stock.)

10. Put in the Cognac and butter during the final minute of cooking, mix thoroughly, and serve instantly.

Milanese Risotto

Serves 6 pax

Ingredients

- 2 pounds beef marrow bones, if possible center-cut from the leg bone
- 2 teaspoons kosher salt
- 2 cups finely chopped onions
- 2 cups Italian short-grain rice, such as Arborio, Carnaroli, or Vialone Nano
- ½ cup freshly grated Grana Padano, plus more for passing
- ½ teaspoon loosely packed saffron threads
- 1 cup dry white wine
- 2 tablespoons extra-virgin olive oil
- 2 tablespoons unsalted butter, cut into pieces
- 6 to 8 cups hot Mixed Meat Stock (chicken or turkey broth could be substituted)

Procedure

1. Heat the stock to a bare simmer in a moderate-sized deep cooking pan. Pour about ½ cup of the stock into a heat-proof cup. Toast the saffron: Drop the strands into the bowl of a metal spoon, separating them a bit. Hold the spoon over a low open flame

2. for just a few seconds, until the aroma is released, then put in the threads to the stock in the cup. Allow them to steep while you start the risotto.

3. Scrape the marrow out of the bones with a sturdy paring knife—do not scrape off any bits of bone. Cut the marrow into little pieces; you should have about ⅓ cup total. Place the olive oil and marrow bits in a moderate-sized Dutch oven on moderate heat. As the marrow melts, mix in the chopped onions and 1 teaspoon salt.

4. Cook while stirring once in a while, for quite a few minutes, until the onions are wilted and just beginning to color; then ladle in ½ cup hot stock from the pot and allow it to simmer until completely vaporized.

5. Put in the rice all at once, raise the heat, and stir for about three minutes, until the grains are toasted but not browned. Pour in the wine, and cook, stirring constantly, until nearly all of the liquid has been absorbed.

6. Pour in 2 cups of the hot stock and stir steadily as the rice absorbs the liquid and starts to release its starch. When you can see the bottom of the pan as you stir, after five minutes or so, ladle in a different couple of cups of stock and the rest of the ½ teaspoon salt.

7. Cook while stirring, until the stock is again nearly fully absorbed. Now pour in the saffron-infused stock together with a cup or so of hot stock from the pot. Cook while stirring, until the liquid is absorbed and the saffron color has spread. Check the risotto: it must be creamy but still firm to the bite.

8. Incorporate more stock if required. When the risotto is fully cooked, remove the heat and whip in the butter pieces, until melted. Mix in the ½ cup of grated cheese, and spoon into warm pasta bowls.

9. Serve instantly, passing additional grated cheese at the table.

Barolo and Carrots Risotto

Ingredients

For the Carrot Purée:

- 3 tablespoons unsalted butter, at room temperature
- Kosher salt
- 3 cups chopped carrots (approximately 2 pounds)
- Pinch of freshly grated nutmeg

For the Risotto:

- ½ cup freshly grated Grana Padano,
- ½ teaspoon kosher salt, or to taste
- 1 cup minced onions
- 2 cups good Barolo wine
- 3 cups Arborio or Carnaroli rice
- 2 tablespoons minced shallots
- 5 tablespoons unsalted butter, cut into bits
- 4 tablespoons extra-virgin olive oil
- 5 cups Chicken Stock or Mixed Meat Stock

Procedure

1. Pour the stock into a small deep cooking pan and bring to a bare simmer. For the carrot purée: Bring a medium deep cooking pan full of salted water to its boiling point.

2. Put in the carrots, and cook until soft, 13 minutes. Drain thoroughly, and pass through a food mill or purée in a food processor. Mix in the butter, nutmeg, and salt to taste. Cover and keep warm.

3. In a moderate-sized Dutch oven or big straight-sided frying pan, heat the olive oil.

4. Put in the onions and shallots, and cook them until golden, stirring frequently, 8 minutes. Put in the rice and stir to coat with the oil. Toast the rice until the edges become translucent, three minutes.

5. Put in ½ cup of the wine, and cook, stirring, until all the wine is absorbed, 4 minutes.

6. Repeat with the rest of the wine in ½-cup batches. Put in ½ cup of the hot stock and the salt. Cook while stirring continuously, until all the stock has been absorbed.

7. Carry on to put in hot stock in small batches— barely sufficient to moisten the rice completely— and cook until each successive batch has been absorbed. Sprinkle with salt.

8. Stir continuously and adjust the level of heat so the rice is simmering very gently while you are putting in the stock, until the rice mixture is creamy but firm to the bite, eighteen minutes from the time the wine was added.

9. Take the pot from the heat. Beat in the butter until completely absorbed, then the grated cheese. Adjust the seasoning with salt, if required, and pepper.

10. To serve: Spread the warm carrot purée over the bottom of six warm shallow bowls. Top with some of the hot risotto.

11. Top each serving with additional grated cheese to taste. Serve instantly.

Truffled Risotto

Serves 6 pax

Ingredients

- ½ teaspoon kosher salt, plus more to taste
- 1 cup minced onions
- 3 ounces fresh white truffle
- Freshly ground black pepper to taste
- 2 tablespoons minced shallots
- ¼ cup freshly grated Grana Padano
- ½ cup dry white wine
- 6 tablespoons unsalted butter, cut into bits
- 2 cups Arborio or Carnaroli rice
- 4 tablespoons extra-virgin olive oil
- 6 cups Chicken Stock

Procedure

1. Brush the truffles meticulously with a vegetable brush to remove as much loose dirt as you can. With a damp paper towel, clean them meticulously.
2. In a small deep cooking pan, heat the stock just to a simmer. In a heavy, wide 3-to4-quart straight-sided frying pan or shallow Dutch oven, heat the olive oil on moderate heat.
3. Put in the onions and shallots, and cook them until golden, stirring frequently, approximately eight minutes. Put in the rice and stir to coat with the oil.
4. Toast the rice until the edges become translucent, approximately three minutes.
5. Pour in the wine and stir until vaporized.
6. Put in ½ cup of the hot stock and the salt. Cook while stirring continuously, until all the stock has been absorbed. Carry on to put in hot stock in small batches—barely sufficient to moisten the rice completely—and cook until each successive batch has been absorbed.

7. Stir continuously and adjust the level of heat so the rice is simmering very gently while you are putting in the stock, until the rice mixture is creamy but firm to the bite.

8. This will take 16 to eighteen minutes from the time the wine is added.

9. Take the frying pan from the heat. Beat in the butter until the butter is melted, then beat in the grated cheese. Adjust the seasoning with salt and pepper.

10. Serve instantly, ladled into warm shallow bowls. Use a truffle slicer or the coarse side of a box grater to shave the truffles over the risotto at the table and let the sublime aroma rise to delight each guest.

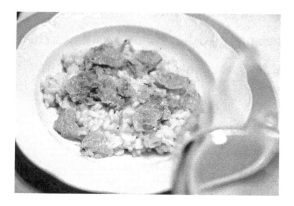

Blossom and Zucchini Risotto

Ingredients

- 1 cup freshly grated Grana Padano
- 1 pound baby zucchini, blossoms still attached
- 1 small onion, finely chopped
- 1 small shallot, finely chopped
- 2 cups Arborio or Carnaroli rice
- 4 tablespoons extra-virgin olive oil
- 6 cups Chicken Stock or water
- ¼ teaspoon saffron threads
- ½ cup dry white wine
- ½ teaspoon kosher salt, plus more to taste
- 6 tablespoons unsalted butter, cut into 6 chunks

Procedure

1. In a moderate-sized deep cooking pan, bring the chicken stock or water to a bare simmer. Separate the blossoms from the zucchini. Cut the zucchini into ¼-inchthick rounds, and the blossoms crosswise into thirds.

2. In a big straight-sided frying pan on moderate heat, heat 2 tablespoons of the olive oil. Once the oil is hot, put in the onion and shallot, and cook, stirring once in a while, until golden, 4 minutes.

3. Put in the zucchini and blossoms, and stir until just wilted, three minutes. Remove zucchini and blossoms to a plate, leaving some of the onion bits behind, and put in the rest of the olive oil to the pot. Soak the saffron threads in ½ cup of the hot stock.

4. Put in the rice and stir to coat in the oil. Toast the rice, without coloring it, for about three minutes.

5. Raise the heat to moderate high, put in the wine, and cook until the wine is reduced away to a glaze, approximately two minutes. Sprinkle with salt.

6. Put in 1 cup of the stock and the saffron and its soaking liquid and regulate the heat so the risotto is simmering.

7. Gradually put in more stock as each addition has been absorbed, stirring all the while, until the rice is firm to the bite and the risotto is creamy, eighteen minutes.

8. For the final five minutes of cooking, return the zucchini to the risotto. (You may not need to use all of the stock.) Stir so the zucchini cooks and amalgamates with the risotto.

9. Take the frying pan from the heat, and beat in the butter, blending it meticulously.

10. Mix in the cheese, tweak the seasoning if required, before you serve.

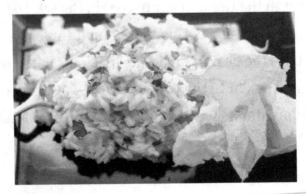

Veggies Risotto

Serves 6 pax

Ingredients

- ½ teaspoon kosher salt, or as required
- 1 cup blanched and peeled fava beans or frozen baby lima beans
- 1 tablespoon minced shallot
- 4 tablespoons unsalted butter, cut into bits
- ½ cup dry white wine
- ½ cup freshly grated Grana Padano
- ½ cup minced scallions, greens included
- 2 cups Arborio or Carnaroli rice
- 5 tablespoons extra-virgin olive oil
- 6 cups Vegetable Stock or Chicken Stock
- 8 ounces broccoli (approximately 1 medium stalk)
- Freshly ground black pepper, to taste

Procedure

1. Bring the stock to a bare simmer in a moderate-sized deep cooking pan. Trim the broccoli florets from the stems, keeping them small enough to fit on a spoon. (You should have approximately 1¼ cups.)

2. Peel the stems, and slice into two-inch pieces. Steam the florets just until bright green, approximately one minute. Steam the stems until super soft, 4 minutes. Reserve the steaming liquid.

3. Move the stems to a blender and process until the desired smoothness is achieved. Scrape out the purée into a small bowl and set the florets and purée aside.

4. If using the baby lima beans, cook them in a small deep cooking pan of boiling salted water for a couple of minutes. Drain them and save for later.

5. Heat the olive oil in a moderate-sized Dutch oven or big straight-sided frying pan on moderate heat. Put in the scallions and shallot, and sauté until translucent, stirring frequently, 4 minutes.

6. Put in the rice and stir to coat with the oil. Toast the rice until the edges become translucent, approximately three minutes. Pour in the wine, and stir thoroughly until it is vaporized, two to three minutes.

7. Put in ½ cup of the hot stock and the salt. Cook while stirring continuously, until all the stock has been absorbed. Carry on to put in hot stock in small batches—barely sufficient to moisten the rice completely—and cook until each successive batch has been absorbed.

8. After the risotto has cooked for about twelve minutes, mix in the broccoli purée and the favas or limas. About three minutes after that, mix in the broccoli florets. Stir and adjust the level of heat so the rice is simmering while you are putting in the stock, until the rice mixture is creamy but firm. This will take 18 minutes from addition of stock.

9. Take the casserole from the heat. Beat in the butter; when it has melted, beat in the grated cheese.

10. Adjust the seasoning with salt, if required, and pepper.

11. Serve instantly, ladled into warm shallow bowls.

Thank you, dear meat lover.

I am glad you accepted my teachings.

These meals have been personally codified in my worldwide trips.

I wanted to share them with you, to let people know more about meat and how to treat it properly.

Now you had come to know about Chicken in all of its shapes, let me give you one more tip.

This manual takes part of an unmissable cookbooks collection.

These meat-based recipes, mixed to all the tastes I met around the world, will give you a complete idea of the possibilities this world offers to us.

You have now the opportunity to add hundreds new elements to your cooking skills knowledge.

Check out the other books!

Dorian Gravy

CPSIA information can be obtained
at www.ICGtesting.com
Printed in the USA
BVHW010421070821
613819BV00024BA/231